Intermittent Fasting

A Comprehensive Manual On The Fasting Lifestyle: A 45-day Regimen
For Optimal Health And Strategies For Effective Weight Management,
Accompanied By Culinary Techniques And Recipe Suggestions

Everette Hensley

TABLE OF CONTENT

The term autophagy denotes a process where a biological entity consumes itself, and it is precisely this mechanism that leads to the decrease in body mass among individuals. Sustained regular eating maintains a state of bodily growth. It harnesses nutrient molecules to produce energy for accomplishing tasks. The cells accumulate the surplus energy within their structure in the guise of adipose tissue. The accumulation of waste materials within the cells of the body occurs as a consequence of internal and external factors. This exerts an influence on your organs, tissues, and ultimately impacts both your overall wellness and body mass.

Nevertheless, once food consumption ceases and fasting begins, the human body initiates a search for alternative energy sources. Consequently, the adipose tissue within the cells undergoes degradation, leading to the liberation of energy. In light of this, autophagy refers to a cellular mechanism wherein damaged components and proteins are eliminated by the body's cells, subsequently undergo recycling, with the ultimate aim of self-renewal.

Autophagy can alternatively be perceived as a cellular mechanism wherein the body's cells eliminate accumulated toxins and subsequently utilize the remnants to synthesize novel substances. A multitude of tissues and organs initiate the phenomenon of autophagy in response to a lack of nourishment.

However, how does the human body determine the appropriate initiation of the autophagy process?

It is imperative to transmit a signal to the organs, prompting them to initiate cellular breakdown in order to generate energy. There are numerous approaches to accomplishing this task. Fasting alone is not the sole catalyst for initiating autophagy within the body. Presented herewith are several alternative methods for achieving weight loss that one may consider.

Exercise

The greater the level of stress exerted on the muscles and cells within your body, the more pronounced the stimulation of the cellular cleansing process will become. Various rigorous forms of physical activity, encompassing activities such as jogging, sprinting, weight training, and physical conditioning, exert a regulatory effect on autophagy through the initiation of stress responses within the human body. In a state of heightened physiological activity, the human body requires a sufficient amount of energy, which is attained through the metabolic process of burning cellular waste.

Cold Showers

Indeed, frigid showers can also facilitate the stimulation of beneficial autophagy within your body. Research has indicated that individuals who engage in swimming activities during the winter period demonstrate elevated capacities for cellular repair and recycling. Hence, incorporating regular cold showers into your routine can contribute to weight loss and promote overall well-being.

Steam Bath

Exposing oneself to elevated temperatures through saunas and steam baths induces thermal stress within the body. The elevated temperature leads to the disintegration and repurposing of malignant and compromised cells.

A visit to a spa facility can offer benefits such as relaxation, rejuvenation, weight loss, and ongoing disease prevention. Additionally, subjecting oneself to intense heat aids in alleviating depression through the natural release of heat shock proteins.

Intermittent Fasting

Certain processes in your body are activated or ceased by indicators. The hormonal levels are amongst the factors at play. Upon commencement of intermittent fasting, the cells are deprived of crucial nutrients. This initiates the secretion of the hormone glucagon within the human body. This hormone functions in counteraction to insulin. While insulin serves to elevate blood glucose levels, glucagon functions to reduce them in order to preserve equilibrium. The two hormones are analogous to the opposing sides of a balancing mechanism.

During the fasting state, insulin levels decrease, leading to an increase in glucagon levels. This rise triggers autophagy. The body receives the signal to initiate the breakdown of stored fats within the body cells in order to restore insulin levels.

Antioxidants

While antioxidants do not directly initiate the process of autophagy within the human body, they have been observed to indirectly contribute to its activation. Foods abundant in antioxidants facilitate the fasting process, thereby promoting a well-regulated and wholesome autophagic response.

Are there any mechanisms that can inhibit autophagy?

Various factors can impede the autophagy process. The primary one is the mechanistic target of rapamycin (mTOR). It inhibits the process of autophagy within your body once an ample supply of nutrients is present within the cells. It exhibits a significant level of sensitivity, as even a minimal intake of 50 calories can enhance mTOR activity.

If dietary fat is ingested, it may not elicit an increase in insulin secretion, thereby potentially maintaining suppression of mTOR levels. However, the presence of significant quantities of ketones and fats will result in the termination of your fasting period.

Please find below a compilation of necessary measures one can adopt to effectively regulate insulin levels and facilitate the cellular waste elimination process within the body:

Green Tea

Coconut Oil

MCT Oil

Ginger compounds

Galangal

Extracts derived from the Reishi mushroom

Black coffee

Acetic acid derived from apples

All of these items have the potential to enhance the process of autophagy within your body.

Does it solely cater to achieving weight loss goals?

Absolutely not. When the cells undergo self-renewal via the process of waste combustion, they exert effects that extend beyond mere weight reduction. Maintaining clean and healthy cells can mitigate the likelihood of disease onset. Various types of cancer, as well as neurodegenerative disorders such as Alzheimer's and Parkinson's, along with metabolic and autoimmune conditions, can be effectively averted by means of autophagy.

It aids in the combat against infectious ailments while also regulating inflammatory responses. Additionally, it has been linked to combatting depression and schizophrenia. Fasting-induced autophagy can be instrumental in promoting overall well-being and mitigating the risk of various medical ailments. It is always beneficial to eliminate the debris in your surroundings and internal sphere. An environment free of dirt and pollutants promotes good health and mitigates occurrences of illness.

Presented here is an inventory outlining the prominent advantages attributed to autophagy, encompassing intracellular as well as extracellular domains.

Increases metabolism

Reduces oxidative stress

Enhances genomic integrity for the prevention of malignancies.

Disposes of bodily waste Removes waste materials from the body Excretes metabolic waste Expels bodily waste products Cleanses the body by eliminating waste

Enhances neuroendocrine equilibrium

Decreases inflammation

Increases lifespan

Removes senescent cells.

Enhances muscular proficiency Enhances muscle function Boosts muscle performance Enhances muscular capabilities Optimizes muscle performance

Does Autophagy Help Women? How?

The ghrelin, also known as the hunger hormone, exhibits a faster rate of increase in women compared to men. Females experience a rapid return of hunger shortly following the consumption of a meal. Their physical systems exhibit a heightened propensity for food intake acceleration, consequently placing them in a state of increased physiological strain to secure additional sources of sustenance. The process of purifying their bodily cells renders them impervious to contracting illnesses and facilitates the enhancement of their immune system.

Does Autophagy Also Contribute to the Process of Age Reversal?

Consider a real-life example. Let us consider the hypothetical scenario in which you possess two automobiles, denoted as X and Y. You appear to have a certain preference for car X, and as a result, you tend to provide it with more diligent maintenance and attention. You engage in daily washing, periodic servicing, and regular refueling of the tank. Conversely, car Y rarely experiences favorable conditions. It serves as an alternative solution for you during the periods when X is unavailable due to maintenance or repairs. The vehicle's fuel tank has not been replenished, it remains encrusted with dirt, and has only undergone a single maintenance check in the span of several years.

Now, based on durability, which vehicle do you believe would exhibit a longer lifespan? Obviously, car X. When one devotes attention to maintaining good health and promptly addressing any necessary repairs, the accumulation of faults and damages can be avoided. Car X is prone to maintaining its pristine condition even after extensive use over the passage of time, while car Y is characterized by an inclination to exhibit operational difficulties relatively early on.

A similar occurrence takes place with the cells within your corporeal composition. The accumulation of non-functional components and cellular waste within the cell impairs your well-being and contributes to the process of aging. However, when individuals consistently engage in recycling and rejuvenating practices, its effects become noticeable on one's complexion. Revitalized and youthful cells contribute to the enhancement of your skin's texture, rendering it more supple and promoting overall vitality.

Autophagy functions as a cellular mechanism for waste degradation and removal. More recent cells eliminate the deceased and unhealthy ones. This results in heightened elimination of senescent cells. Autophagy decelerates the aging process within the body, thereby imparting a youthful and robust appearance over an extended duration.

What is the Mechanism by Which the Body Undergoes Renewal Through Autophagy?

Even the most minute details hold significance, particularly when it pertains to the process of aging, as those minor aspects take precedence. Cells are the fundamental components responsible for maintaining both one's health and susceptibility to illness. They store and provide energy, facilitate oxygen transportation, and perform essential functions for the human body. Furthermore, they are the ones responsible for preserving your youthfulness both internally and externally.

Allow us to gain comprehension of the mechanics behind this process. The cells within your body are in a ceaseless state of activity, thereby subjecting them to a considerable amount of physical strain and deterioration. The excessively employed cells ultimately halt their functionality, thereby rendering them ineffectual. In such instances, the proliferation of fresh and robust cells is likewise impeded by the presence of non-functional cells.

These depleted cells are commonly referred to as senescent cells. A senescent cell is a viable cellular entity, albeit its functionality does not contribute to the preservation of an individual's well-being. Furthermore, not only do they fail to contribute to any physiological processes, but they also inhibit the formation of new cells within the body. Throughout the course of time, the aging cells relentlessly amass within the human body. They exclusively carry out fundamental actions, impede the formation of fresh cells, and facilitate the onset of inflammation. One of the most detrimental aspects for women is that they accelerate the aging process of the adjacent cells.

Autophagy facilitates the removal of impaired cells, thus creating a favorable environment for the emergence of rejuvenated cells. You retain youthfulness, robust health, and vitality over an extended duration. Hence, striving to eliminate the waste within your body cells is a commendable endeavor for you to undertake.

Cultivating wholesome practices in one's life is an effective means of leading a virtuous existence. An unkempt dwelling is universally disliked, whereas a meticulously maintained residence, adorned with pristine furnishings, garners favor from both its occupants and observers alike. Autophagy is a cellular process that facilitates the removal of outdated components within a living organism, allowing for the replenishment of vital resources.

***

Research on the effects of intermittent fasting.

It may come as a surprise to you that the majority of us inherently practice fasting daily during our sleeping hours. You may consider prolonging the inherent period of fasting for a slightly longer duration. As an illustration, one may choose to forgo breakfast and instead commence their first meal at noon, concluding with their final meal at 8 pm. This practice would constitute a variation of intermittent fasting.

With this approach, an individual essentially observes a fasting duration of sixteen hours on a daily basis, followed by a limited feeding window of eight hours. This particular style of fasting, commonly referred to as the 16/8 method, stands out as one of the prevailing choices within the realm of intermittent fasting.

Contrary to your current assumptions, it should be noted that intermittent fasting is in fact more manageable than anticipated. Minimal planning is required, and a plethora of individuals who have adhered to this dietary regimen have frequently attested to experiencing enhanced well-being and heightened vitality during periods of food abstinence. Initially, one may experience some difficulty in managing hunger, but it won't be long before the body acclimates and adapts to the new circumstance.

Why fast?

The subsequent inquiry that may arise pertains to the rationale behind considering fasting as a viable course of action. Throughout history, human beings have consistently engaged in cycles of fasting for prolonged periods. On certain occasions, they resorted to this course of action out of necessity, as a result of their inability to procure sustenance. Furthermore, on certain occasions, fasting was also observed for religious purposes. Religious practices such as Buddhism, Christianity, and Islam prescribe various forms of abstaining from food, commonly known as fasting. Furthermore, it is customary to abstain from eating during periods of illness.

Despite fasting occasionally being associated with negativity, it is undeniable that fasting is a completely natural phenomenon. Indeed, our physiological systems are adequately equipped to cope with periods of food deprivation. There are a considerable number of physiological processes within the human body that undergo alterations during a period of fasting. This phenomenon facilitates the sustenance of our bodies amidst periods characterized by scarcity of resources.

During periods of fasting, there is a notable decrease in insulin and blood sugar levels, along with a considerable elevation of a hormone called the human growth hormone. Although initially employed during times of food scarcity, this practice has evolved to aid in weight reduction of individuals. Through the practice of fasting, the process of fat burning is facilitated, streamlined, and highly efficacious.

Certain individuals opt to embark on a period of fasting as it has the potential to enhance their metabolic functions. This form of fasting is beneficial for enhancing a wide range of health disorders and afflictions. Moreover, there exists evidence substantiating the notion that practicing intermittent fasting has the potential to extend one's lifespan. Research indicates that rodents were able to increase their lifespan through the practice of intermittent fasting.

Alternative: "Additional studies have demonstrated that fasting can confer safeguarding effects against a range of ailments, inclusive of but not limited to Alzheimer's disease, cancer, type-2 diabetes, and heart disease." Additionally, some individuals opt for intermittent fasting as it aligns conveniently with their lifestyle. Fasting has proven to be a highly efficacious technique for enhancing one's life. For example, as the number of meals you need to prepare decreases, your life will become more streamlined.

What is the underlying mechanism behind the efficacy of intermittent fasting?

Upon commencing intermittent fasting, it is expected that your caloric intake will remain unchanged, although instead of distributing your meals evenly throughout the day, you will consume larger meals within a condensed time period. As an illustration, instead of consuming 3 to 4 meals throughout the day, it can be suggested to partake in a single substantial meal at 11 am, followed by another sizeable meal at 6 pm. During the period between 11 am and 6 pm, abstain from eating any meals. Furthermore, after 6 pm, refrain from consuming any meals until 11 am the following day. This represents merely a singular approach to intermittent fasting, with the subsequent chapters in this book aiming to elucidate alternative methodologies. Nevertheless, it is essential to grasp the underlying principles behind the efficacy of this approach.

Intermittent fasting is a modality employed by a substantial number of bodybuilders, athletes, and fitness enthusiasts in order to effectively maintain considerable levels of muscle mass and simultaneously minimize their body fat percentage. It is a straightforward approach that enables individuals to indulge in their preferred foods while simultaneously facilitating the reduction of body fat and the acquisition or preservation of muscle mass. Intermittent fasting can be implemented on a temporary or permanent basis, however, the optimal outcomes are achieved by incorporating this approach as a habitual part of your everyday routine.

Despite the potentially alarming connotations associated with the term "fasting," it is important to note that intermittent fasting does not involve depriving oneself of sustenance. In order to comprehend the underlying concepts of effective intermittent fasting, it is imperative to initially delve into the two distinct physiological states of digestion that the human body undergoes, namely the fed state and the fasting state.

During a span of three to five hours following the consumption of a meal, the body enters a physiological phase referred to as the "fed state." Amid this period, the secretion of insulin escalates to facilitate the absorption and digestion of the ingested food. When the levels of insulin in your body are elevated, the process of fat burning becomes considerably challenging. Insulin is a hormone secreted by the pancreas in order to maintain glycemic control in the circulatory system. Despite its primary function being regulation, insulin is classified as a storage hormone. Elevated insulin levels lead to the utilization of ingested food for energy instead of stored fat, thus hindering weight loss.

Once the period of three to five hours has elapsed, your body completes the digestion of the meal and transitions into the post-absorptive phase. The duration of the post-absorptive state ranges from 8 to 12 hours. Subsequent to this temporal interval, your body transitions into the state of fasting. Given that your body has fully undergone the digestion process at this juncture, the levels of insulin in your system are minimal, thereby facilitating easy access to your stored fat for the purpose of oxidation.

During the state of fasting, the body depletes its food reserves, leading to the utilization of stored fat for energy generation. Intermittent fasting facilitates the attainment of an enhanced state of fat metabolism that would typically be achieved through a conventional eating regimen of three meals per day. This singular factor is solely responsible for the notable expeditious outcomes observed by numerous individuals practicing intermittent fasting, even in the absence of alterations to their habitual exercise regimens, food quantity, or dietary content. They are merely altering the temporal and sequential aspects of their dietary consumption.

When commencing an intermittent fasting regimen, there may be a period of adjustment required to establish a routine. Do not allow yourself to become disheartened! In the event of a misstep, simply resume your intermittent fasting routine as soon as you are able. Refrain from engaging in self-criticism or experiencing feelings of remorse. Engaging in detrimental self-dialogue will merely extend the period of time it takes for you to return to your habitual routine. Adopting a new way of living necessitates deliberate commitment, and it is not expected that you will flawlessly achieve it immediately. If one is not accustomed to extended periods of abstaining from food, intermittent fasting may require an adjustment period. Provided that you select an appropriate approach for yourself, maintain your concentration, and adopt an optimistic mindset, mastery of the task will swiftly ensue.

In contrast to certain alternative diet plans you may choose to follow, the intermittent fasting regimen is highly effective. It leverages the functionality of your body to its benefit, facilitating effective weight loss. It is common to experience a mild sense of apprehension upon learning about the practice of fasting. One may postulate that an extended period of abstinence from food is required (although it is improbable for individuals to possess the fortitude necessary to forgo sustenance for such an extended duration, even when motivated to achieve weight loss), resulting in perceived hardship.

Intermittent fasting deviates from common expectations. Not only does enduring a prolonged fast pose significant challenges, but it also has detrimental effects on the body. If an individual sustains an extended period of fasting, their body may frequently enter a state of metabolic adaptation known as starvation mode. It presupposes a context characterized by scarcity of sustenance, wherein the body endeavors to conserve calories by retaining fat reserves for prolonged periods. This implies that not solely are you experiencing hunger, but you are also negating the opportunity to accomplish weight loss.

There is no need for excessive concern regarding the efficacy of this intermittent fasting approach during periods of metabolic starvation. The intermittent fasting method proves efficacious as it prevents prolonged fasting that could trigger a state of starvation in the body, consequently inhibiting weight loss. On the contrary, it will ensure that the duration of the fast is sufficient to facilitate an acceleration of the metabolic rate.

Through the implementation of intermittent fasting, it will become evident that refraining from the consumption of food for several hours (typically no longer than approximately 24 hours) will not prompt the body to immediately enter a state of starvation. Instead, it will expend the calories that are accessible. If an individual consumes an appropriate caloric intake, the body will proceed to utilize the accumulated fat reserves as a source of energy. Consequently, by adhering to an intermittent fasting regimen, you compel your body to incinerate additional fat with minimal exertion.

EMPIRICAL INVESTIGATION INTO THE PHENOMENON OF INTERMITTENT FASTING

You have acquired considerable knowledge regarding Intermittent Fasting thus far; however, it is plausible that you have yet to grasp the underlying mechanisms behind its efficacy concerning dietary practices and overall well-being. This chapter serves as an elucidating remedy for such perplexity! You will acquire knowledge about the impact of Intermittent Fasting on the human body, its correlation with diabetes, heart health, aging, and ultimately, its effects on the female physiology. Upon the completion of this chapter, it is anticipated that you will possess a comprehensive understanding of IF, in addition to being cognizant of a few possible intricacies that may arise.

The Impact of Intermittent Fasting on the Human Body

When experiencing hunger, the functioning of two pivotal hormones, namely leptin and ghrelin, exert a significant influence on the body. Intermittent Fasting considerably impacts the regulation of these hormones. Under ordinary circumstances, it is customary for leptin to suppress feelings of hunger, whereas ghrelin elicits sensations of hunger in individuals. Leptin is produced and released by adipocytes distributed across the body, whereas ghrelin is exclusively synthesized within the stomach lining. In tandem, leptin and ghrelin engage in effective communication with the hypothalamus of the brain, regulating the initiation and cessation of food intake. During intermittent fasting, there is a reduction in the frequency of hormone release, leading to a distinct alteration in the body's perception of hunger and satiety.

Furthermore, in the context of appetite regulation and satiety, insulin constitutes another pivotal hormone. The pancreas is responsible for the secretion of insulin, which plays a vital role in the regulation of blood glucose levels. In essence, the individual's weight is significantly influenced by varying levels of insulin. Insufficient insulin levels impair weight maintenance. Excessive insulin levels significantly impede weight loss efforts. Although the desire is for lower insulin levels, it is essential to maintain a proper equilibrium, as excessively low levels of insulin can be detrimental to the body due to the significant role that glucose (or blood sugar) plays in providing energy to the body.

An additional determinant of an individual's appetite and weight loss status is the functioning of their thyroid gland. In the event of thyroid hyperactivity, metabolic processes will be accelerated, resulting in consequential impacts on energy levels, overall health, and body weight. On the contrary, a hypothyroid condition will have an inhibitory effect on metabolism, energy levels, overall health, and will consequently lead to weight gain.

Ultimately, Intermittent Fasting imparts an impact on an individual's body weight through modulation of the production of these three vital hormones and synergistically leveraging the inherent capabilities of the thyroid gland. In essence, individuals who engage in intermittent fasting will induce a less frequent release of these hormones (or a more regular release in the case of obesity or diabetes) owing to the reduced frequency of their eating patterns. Over time, the effects of the thyroid should reach equilibrium as a result of this modified dietary regimen.

The Relationship Between IF and Diabetes

For individuals afflicted with diabetes, Intermittent Fasting presents both potential hazards and remarkable advantages. Individuals suffering from diabetes exhibit modified insulin levels in comparison to those who do not have the condition, attributable to the presence of insulin resistance within their physiological systems. Individuals with Type 1 diabetes have an inability to produce insulin. Administration of insulin on a daily basis is necessary for them to sustain the requisite vitality and liveliness in their lives. Individuals diagnosed with Type 2 diabetes exhibit limited production of insulin or inefficiency in the utilization of insulin within their bodies.

With the introduction of these modified iterations of insulin, the body lacks the means to regulate blood sugar levels, resulting in a perpetual presence of glucose in the bloodstream, without the ability to be effectively utilized by cells for natural and physical energy. The elevated blood glucose level can lead to further complications for the individual in the long run; however, there is no legitimate remedy apart from the daily administration of insulin.

Intermittent fasting, when properly implemented in the lives of individuals with diabetes (whose diabetic conditions are not severe), can offer a transient remedy. When individuals afflicted with diabetes engage in daily IF, incorporating only a few fasting hours per day, they exhibit amelioration in terms of weight, blood sugar levels, and glycemic status. It is not advisable for these individuals to forgo complete meals or engage in prolonged periods of fasting. Additionally, it is not advisable for individuals in this category to strictly adhere to a diet while practicing intermittent fasting. Alternatively, adopting the approach of reducing food portions and minimizing the consumption of snacks in between meals yields more favorable results.

The Impact of IF on Cardiovascular Health

Cardiovascular health is a complex matter in contemporary society. We all aspire to maintain good health and prosper, yet our dietary choices and lifestyle pursuits frequently diverge from these aspirations, resulting in prioritization of more immediate gratification. Consequently, a substantial number of our hearts are not in optimal condition. Heart disease remains the leading cause of mortality worldwide in contemporary times. Nevertheless, the incorporation of Intermittent Fasting into an individual's lifestyle can significantly mitigate these risks, as it has the potential to decrease the likelihood of cardiovascular ailments.

For instance, recent empirical investigations on animals have demonstrated that the implementation of Intermittent Fasting yields enhancements in multiple risk indicators associated with cardiovascular illness. Some examples of these enhancements encompass decreased cholesterol levels, mitigated inflammation within the body, regulated blood sugar levels, and diminished blood pressure. Fundamentally, intermittent fasting does not possess the ability to cure heart disease; however, it does possess the potential to mitigate various risk factors inherent in one's physiological state, whether they are aware of them or not.

In essence, provided that one incorporates the replenishment of electrolytes into their Intermittent Fasting routine, there is absolutely no inherent risk to the cardiovascular system. There exists solely the capacity for expansion, fortification, and enhancement. Nevertheless, in the absence of proper restoration of electrolytes, there remains the potential for cardiac arrhythmias in individuals pursuing intermittent fasting. The cardiac system necessitates electrolytes for maintaining its stability and efficiency. Hence, incorporating a small amount of salt into your water intake would be greatly appreciated by your heart.

The Intersection of IF and the Aging Process

Individuals often engage in discussions about how Intermittent Fasting possesses the ability to counteract the aging process, and it is an accurate assertion. However, the challenge lies in effectively expounding upon the scientific principles that underlie the mentioned phenomenon. The potential for countering the effects of aging associated with Intermittent Fasting primarily pertains to two aspects: 1) cognitive function and 2) the entirety of the body, through a process known as "autophagy."

In general, Intermittent Fasting facilitates the healing of the body by effectively revitalizing the cells. By adhering to an eating schedule or timing that imposes a limited caloric intake, the cells of the body are able to operate with reduced constraints and ambiguity, thereby facilitating enhanced energy production for bodily functions. Essentially, the cells operate with enhanced efficiency, enabling the body to effectively utilize fat and oxygen for the optimal function of organs and blood. Consequently, individuals experience an extended lifespan and heightened feelings of rejuvenation.

Concerning the aforementioned two specific instances, there has been substantial evidence to support the notion that Intermittent Fasting effectively maintains and enhances cognitive abilities. It enhances overall cognitive functioning and memory capacity, while also fostering astuteness, acuity, and prompt and lucid thinking in the present. Moreover, Intermittent Fasting also promotes cellular fitness and agility through autophagy, which is initiated by IF. This biological process prompts the cells to undergo self-cleansing and eliminate any accumulated waste materials that could impede their functionality. By gradually implementing limitations on your eating timeframe on a daily or weekly basis, you can experience an enhancement in cognitive abilities and achieve physical preparedness to face any challenge.

The Intersection of IF and the Female Anatomy

Intermittent Fasting necessitates a distinct approach compared to conventional dietary methods, hence its more common designation as a lifestyle. Moreover, this disparity implies that the impacts of intermittent fasting on the female physique diverge slightly from those of a conventional diet. As an illustration, adhering to a dietary regimen tends to yield consistent weight loss results for the majority, whereas the implementation of intermittent fasting presents a more intricate and notably less dependable process, particularly for women.

The physiological requirements of the female physique, which is naturally equipped for childbirth, are subject to modification under an eating regimen incorporating Intermittent Fasting. Due to a decreased secretion of hormones that regulate appetite and satiety in women, there is a concurrent reduction in adipose tissue accumulation as well as diminished potential for fertility in their subsequent reproductive endeavors. When combined with a rigorously controlled dietary regimen that entails calorie counting or fat restriction, Intermittent Fasting may pose risks for females across various age groups.

There remains a significant prospect for women who desire to incorporate Intermittent Fasting into their routine.

Simply adhere to these four guidelines in order to ensure a health-conscious approach that considers the well-being of both your body and the potential offspring. Initially, it is imperative to establish a strong connection with one's physical form. It is imperative to be highly cognizant of any abnormalities or discrepancies in one's internal state, encompassing physical, emotional, and mental aspects. This is particularly crucial, given the significant consequences in terms of hormone balance and reproductive health.

Furthermore, exert diligent endeavor to maintain a keen awareness of your body's cycles and duly take note when irregularities manifest. Lacking proper understanding of your menstrual cycle, you potentially expose yourself to prolonged disruptions in its regularity. This modification may appear insignificant, nevertheless it has the potential to substantially impact various facets of your physiological well-being and your potential for raising offspring.

Furthermore, it is advised against attempting to simultaneously integrate stringent dietary practices with the application of Intermittent Fasting. I understand your desire to achieve a healthy, fit, and lean physique. However, it is crucial to ensure an adequate intake of fats and calories, taking into account how your body utilizes these essential nutrients at optimal levels.

Lastly, ensure that you are not engaging in excessively vigorous exercise during the initial phase of your transition to Intermittent Fasting. If you have been engaged in the practice of intermittent fasting as a long-term lifestyle, you are certainly encouraged to reintroduce physical fitness and exercise into your regimen. However, it is important to note that combining two vigorous activities simultaneously can pose a significant risk to the female physiology. I comprehend the desire to reduce weight and maintain good health; nevertheless, it is crucial to ensure that you do not excessively eliminate substances from your body simultaneously.

Key Information Regarding Intermittent Fasting

While intermittent fasting offers numerous advantages, it does encounter certain criticisms. As an illustration, certain individuals hold the notion that fasting poses risks due to its restriction of calorie intake, heightened sensation of hunger, or hindrance to weight loss by triggering the body's starvation response. Nevertheless, such beliefs are all fallacies, considering that fasting has been adopted for centuries across the globe as a means to maintain good health. It is advisable to seek guidance from a medical professional regarding your dietary plans to ascertain their suitability for you, much like any other diet.

Binge eating is specifically excluded" "It does not encompass binge eating" "Binge eating is not part of it

Numerous critics contend that individuals engaged in dieting may partake in excessive eating as an attempt to compensate for the "lost" calories subsequent to a period of fasting. However, this assertion does not hold true for the majority of individuals. The objective of fasting is to acquire the skill to regulate one's dietary patterns, resulting in reduced caloric intake and subsequent weight loss. Whereas one might engage in excessive eating due to hunger on alternative diets, the objective of intermittent fasting is to abstain from food for specific periods and demonstrate self-mastery to maintain adherence. Please be aware that it is possible to modify the manner in which you observe fasting to align with your personal requirements. If you have concerns about facing difficulties, consider initially fasting for shorter durations and gradually extending the duration as you become more at ease.

Starvation

The purpose of this dietary regimen is to educate the mind to discern the genuine requirements of the body. During fasting, you are not depriving yourself of sustenance; rather, you are instructing your body about its ability to endure periods of abstinence from food. Moreover, through the establishment of authority over one's eating patterns, it is conceivable to mitigate the occurrence of stress-induced eating, a commonly observed coping mechanism. After extended adherence to intermittent fasting, individuals are expected to adopt a more wholesome perspective towards food, prioritizing their bodily sustenance rather than resorting to emotional coping mechanisms.

Difficult to comprehend

Certain critics express concerns regarding the potential challenges associated with adhering to this dietary regimen. Although this may hold true initially, it is important to bear in mind that this phenomenon occurs due to the process of altering one's psychological perception towards food. During this period, your body will signal a desire for sugary sustenance or increased intake to appease your cravings. Nevertheless, as you adapt to the dietary regimen, it will progressively become more manageable as you cultivate mastery over your consumption patterns.

The Effects of Intermittent Fasting on Menopause

Menopause poses significant challenges for women, and those in the post-menopausal phase must undergo substantial adjustments without the added concern of exacerbating their symptoms through the incorporation of a fasting regimen into their daily routines. The decline in estrogen levels in the body leads to alterations in fat distribution, resulting in the accumulation of fat cells in previously unaffected regions and, in certain instances, causing unanticipated increases in body weight.

It is widely acknowledged among fitness and health experts that menopausal and post-menopausal women derive the greatest health and wellness advantages from the practice of Intermittent Fasting compared to individuals of other genders or age groups. Research findings indicate that individuals who have reached menopause, particularly post-menopausal women, demonstrate a tendency to experience weight loss at a rate that is approximately twice as high as that observed in individuals of the same sex and similar fasting regimens.

One rationale behind this phenomenon is that post-menopausal women demonstrate a higher propensity to adhere to their dietary restrictions and fasting regimen as compared to their pre-menopausal counterparts, as supported by statistical evidence.

Additionally, women within this group are reaching the culmination or conclusion of their menstrual cycles, leading the body to recognize that there is no longer a necessity to allocate calories towards the reproductive processes. Following menopause, the likelihood of experiencing hormonal imbalances decreases as the body effectively adjusts to diminished estrogen levels. Consequently, it becomes more convenient to adapt to a calorie-restricted diet and a more demanding Intermittent Fasting approach.

Instances in Which Women Should Avoid Experimenting with Intermittent Fasting

While it is encouraged for women to capitalize on the multitude of advantages presented by Intermittent Fasting, it is important to acknowledge that there exist a few exceptions and specific situations in which women should adhere to their customary calorie intake.

Pregnancy is among these aforementioned circumstances. Females who are currently expecting or attempting to conceive should refrain from engaging in any form of fasting. Indeed, professionals and nutrition experts advise that pregnant females incorporate an additional 300 to 500 calories into their usual dietary intake during the latter stages of their second and third trimesters. Additionally, pregnant women encounter the greatest variations in their crucial blood parameters during this period. As an illustration, it is noteworthy that a majority of women commonly experience abrupt decreases in blood pressure and blood sugar levels throughout pregnancy, irrespective of their dietary fasting practices or adherence to the recommended daily caloric intake.

Several health hazards associated with fasting during pregnancy include:

There has been an elevation in the likelihood of preterm delivery.

Enhances the likelihood of suboptimal neonatal weight outcomes

Insufficient essential nutrients for both the mother and the child.

Increased likelihood of health complications for the mother both during and following pregnancy.

Additionally, there have been reports postulating that engaging in fasting practices throughout pregnancy may result in future health complications for the offspring. However, it should be noted that sufficient substantiating evidence to confirm this hypothesis is presently lacking. Ultimately, a primary motivation for individuals adopting Intermittent Fasting is weight reduction, a pursuit that should not be prioritized by expectant women during pregnancy.

Armed with this information, it is not beyond the realm of possibility for expectant women to maintain their fast during pregnancy. However, it is regarded as safe only for those who have previously observed fasting for a minimum duration of two years prior to conceiving. Individuals who have been practicing fasting for an extended period, to the extent that it has become deeply ingrained, and have concerns about the potential impact of calorie intake increment on their body, are advised to consult with their physician to determine the optimal course of action.

It is recommended that pregnant women refrain from consuming refined sugars and processed foods, instead directing their dietary intake towards protein-rich and nutrient-dense carbohydrates, in order to adequately support maternal and fetal health.

Children within a specific age range ought to avoid engaging in fasting as well. During early childhood, it is essential for children to consume an adequate amount of vitamins and nutrients in order to develop into physically robust and healthy individuals. Children exhibit elevated metabolic rates, thus it is crucial to ensure they attain the prescribed daily caloric intake in order to mitigate potential health complications.

It is advised that adolescent females who are either below the age of pubescence or currently experiencing puberty refrain from partaking in fasting. During this period, women are most susceptible to experiencing hormone imbalance, which can significantly impact their physiological well-being. Abstaining from food intake during the period of adolescence can give rise to potential complications concerning a woman's reproductive capacity and her capacity to maintain appropriate levels of estrogen throughout her lifespan.

Individuals who already exhibit a deficiency in body weight or possess a history of eating disorders are advised to abstain from engaging in any form of fasting. Deliberately abstaining from eating, even for brief intervals, has the potential to arouse detrimental patterns and tendencies that are psychologically associated with conditions such as anorexia and bulimia. Individuals who face challenges in maintaining a healthy weight suitable for their age and physique will not derive advantages from the practice of Intermittent Fasting, as their bodies possess minimal excess weight to eliminate and are generally already operating under conditions resembling a survival mode. These individuals are additionally advised to abstain from practicing Intermittent Fasting, in order to prevent exacerbating their calorie intake restrictions and potentially heightening their susceptibility to health complications.

Green Smoothie

Ingredients:

- 2 cups coconut milk
- 2 cups chard, spinach or kale, discard hard stems and ribs, torn
- 2 avocados, peeled, pitted, cubed
- ½ cup blueberries
- 2 tbsp chia seeds

Method:

1. Add all the ingredients in a blender and blend until smooth.

2. Pour into glasses and serve.

IF offers numerous advantages, with the most evident outcomes being the reduction of body fat and the enhancement of muscle definition or muscle development. The subsequent paragraphs outline the recognized advantages identified in diverse research studies:

The extension of Telomeres is observed in the context of Interferon (IF) treatment.

What impact does this have? Telomeres serve as protective caps at the termini of an individual's chromosomes. Endeavor to draw a comparison between it and the plastic casings found on the terminus of shoelaces. From a technical standpoint, a direct correlation exists between the length of an individual's telomeres and their potential life expectancy. The elongation of telomeres can occur through dietary restriction. Therefore, the phrase "eat-fast-and live longer" is frequently attributed to intermittent fasting (IF) or other fasting methods.

Intermittent fasting provides a respite for the digestive system.

Given that humans consume food on a regular basis, the digestive system remains in a constant state of activity. The consumption of a wide range of food items, including processed food, can potentially result in gastrointestinal complications. Hence, the act of fasting, specifically intermittent fasting (IF), can be likened to granting respite to the digestive system from its strenuous daily duties. You are permitting it to undergo a period of relaxation and purification.

▢ Cellular autophagy.

This is the physiological mechanism by which the organism undergoes protein recycling. Cellular repair and turnover also take place during this stage. Consider it as a process where cells engage in self-renewal and self-repair, leading to the generation of fresh cells.

Enhanced generation of Ketones.

Ketones are synthesized as a result of the metabolism of adipose tissues utilized by the body as a source of energy, in contrast to the utilization of glucose. Additionally, they assist in curbing one's appetite. Throughout the process of intermittent fasting (IF), an increased quantity of ketones is synthesized, which effectively assist in suppressing the typical sensations of hunger experienced during periods of abstaining from food.

⬜ Fat Burning

Following the consumption of food, the human body initiates the secretion of insulin in order to maintain blood glucose levels within a safe range. The primary function of insulin is to facilitate the movement of surplus sugar, known as glucose, from the bloodstream to various sites within the body, such as the muscles, liver, or adipose tissues, where it is stored for future use. In addition to facilitating glucose removal from the bloodstream, insulin also contributes to heightened adipose tissue accumulation. Reconsider your actions, for each instance of eating, you are enabling your body to secrete a hormone that promotes the storage of fat.

Enhances the production of hormones and enzymes that promote the breakdown of fats.

The hormone somatropin, commonly referred to as growth hormone, has the ability to elevate glucose levels while simultaneously promoting the utilization of stored adipose tissue. During the period of fasting, there is an increased level of activity exhibited by the growth hormones, resulting in a proportional elevation in the rate of fat oxidation, effectively doubling the amount of fats metabolized. In addition, IF enhances the functioning of Hormone Sensitive Lipase (HSL) in adipose tissue and Lipoprotein Lipase (LPL) in muscle tissue. The integration of the HSL and LPL mechanisms maximizes the body's ability to metabolize fat. The adipose tissue hormone-sensitive lipase (HSL) assumes responsibility for the liberation of adipocytes that will be utilized by the body as a source of energy. The muscle tissue releases the enzyme LPL, which signals the muscles to metabolize the fat as a source of energy.)

⦿ Metabolism

In retrospect, during prehistoric eras, individuals did not possess the privilege of partaking in regular and dependable sustenance. They consumed meals during the periods of food availability, and resorted to intermittent fasting during the periods of food unavailability. In reality, the human body does not inherently require a perpetual state of nourishment as it has the capacity to naturally tap into its reservoirs of adipose tissue.

⬚ IF promotes simplicity

Given that an individual is relieved from the task of deciding the content of their breakfast or other meals throughout the day, they are afforded the opportunity to allocate their time and attention towards matters of greater significance. Intermittent fasting (IF) enhances physical strength, diminishes body fat, and encourages a salubrious way of living, all accomplished by consuming only one or two meals daily instead of the customary three or four meals.

According to scholarly investigations, a significant majority of individuals who have experimented with intermittent fasting or incorporated it into their daily routine have demonstrated a considerable level of deliberation and value towards their dietary choices. They became aware that consuming food is the intersection of voluntary decision-making and a bestowed advantage. They acquired knowledge regarding the underlying factors contributing to their hunger and the selection of their food.

Numerous individuals who experimented with intermittent fasting for a single day expressed that they did not experience a sense of deprivation throughout the fasting interval. There exist more stringent IF programs that impose limitations on the quantity of food intake, however, there are no specific provisions that prohibit the consumption of any particular food item.

ACQUIRE KNOWLEDGE REGARDING THE DIVERSE CATEGORIES OF FASTING AND DETERMINE THE OPTIMAL CHOICE FOR YOUR NEEDS

At this juncture, it is conceivable that you have embraced the practice of fasting. Upon examination of the empirical evidence supporting these findings, one becomes cognizant of their potential to facilitate weight loss while concurrently combating and averting various ailments. Nevertheless, do you find yourself pondering about its practical application in reality? Abstaining from food is not merely the sole component of fasting, as there exist numerous strategies that can be employed to effectively aid your physical well-being during this practice. In order for your body to experience the advantages of fasting, it is necessary to subject your body to specific forms of physiological stress. The focus does not lie in experiencing stress in professional or personal life, rather it pertains to deliberately subjecting one's cells to stress during specific periods to activate internal mechanisms. It is imperative to acknowledge that stress does not always induce a sense of comfort, as well. Particularly during the initial stages, you might encounter a sense of unease in the undertaking. Later on, you will acquire knowledge regarding strategies for surmounting certain discomforts. However, acknowledging their existence and anticipating their occurrence will enable you to make more effective preparations.

Fasting is intended to facilitate the purification of the body by enabling it to eliminate toxins and accumulated waste. This implies the necessity of curbing your consumption of food and beverages for a designated duration. During a period of fasting, only water is permitted for consumption. If an individual adheres to an alternative program of purification that incorporates substances other than water into their system, it can be inferred that said program does not genuinely strive to eliminate all cellular toxins in order to restore and maintain one's well-being. Rather than expending funds on extravagant beverage blends or meal packages, consider forgoing a meal or two, or even three, on certain days of the week to initiate a detoxification process within your body. Currently, your body does not possess conscious contentment. Your body has developed a strong dependence on the continuous supply of glucose that you provide. Remove that, and it becomes slightly irritable. This is characterized by the occurrence of fatigue, irritability, cognitive impairment, and analogous manifestations. Nevertheless, the advantages are occurring internally and will ultimately manifest themselves across all levels, provided that sufficient time is allowed for the process to unfold. In addition, one can derive enduring benefits from this. Fasting can be practiced in a discontinuous manner, over an extended period, or on alternating days.

The determination of the optimal fasting regimen for oneself is contingent upon several factors, including individual objectives, present state of health, and prevailing lifestyle. It is of utmost importance that you familiarize yourself with the various forms of fasting and understand how they can be incorporated into your lifestyle.

Subsequently, you may determine your preferred point of commencement, desired destination, and the strategies you intend to employ in order to sustain its progress in the foreseeable future. Prior to reaching that point, initiate the process by delineating your objectives. In the subsequent segment, kindly enumerate significant factors, such as your intended objectives associated with the practice of fasting. Are the goals encompassed as follows: weight reduction, disease prevention, enhancement of overall welfare, or the management of illness? Please record your response or responses in the space provided below:

Now that you have gained clarity regarding your objectives, kindly spare a moment to contemplate on your overall well-being. Are you presently afflicted with any form of ailment or medical condition? Are you collaborating with a healthcare provider to alleviate your illness or infection? Alternatively, are you in good overall health and not currently prescribed medication or under the care of a medical professional? Please provide a written account of your current state of health below:

Prior to implementing your fasting plans, it is imperative that you consult and communicate with your healthcare professionals, especially if you are currently managing a medical condition. Ensure that you establish precise objectives with them and elucidate the rationale behind your decision to undertake fasting as a means to accomplish those goals. Subsequently, expound upon the strategies and approaches proposed by your medical team in order to realistically achieve the set objectives for your situation. If you possess a state of overall physical well-being, it is advisable to consult with your healthcare provider prior to embarking on a new regimen to improve your lifestyle.

Prior to determining the optimal fasting regimen, it is vital to deliberate upon your lifestyle. This encompasses your present dietary patterns, encompassing the timing of your meals, the quantity of food consumed, and the usual composition of your meals. Additionally, assess your frequency of dining out in comparison to preparing the majority of your meals at home. Are you capable of preparing your own meals, or do you rely on dining out? Additionally, please review your itinerary. Do you adhere to a relatively consistent routine, or does your schedule frequently undergo variations? Could you please provide some insight into the frequency with which you engage in business meals or dinners with clients or individuals? Do you engage in social activities, such as attending gatherings with colleagues or acquaintances for the purpose of having beverages and participating in happy hour, during weekends or evenings? Ascertain your habitual way of living. Kindly provide your review in the space provided:

Now that you have acquired knowledge about your objectives, present state of health, and daily routine, you can commence the process of analyzing various forms of fasting. Please keep in mind: fasting should not be perceived as a "diet" where there are specific food restrictions or labeling certain foods as "bad" that need to be avoided. Instead, it could be seen as an alternative dining timetable. Consequently, you have the opportunity to examine your timetable and ascertain the most suitable eating schedule that aligns with your routine. Nevertheless, one can alternatively employ their goals as a means to determine the utilization of this schedule in order to achieve those goals and estimate the duration required.

Intermittent Fasting

One of the prevailing modes of intermittent fasting worthy of consideration is the 16/8 protocol. This implies that you opt for a sixteen-hour fasting period, with a designated eight-hour window solely allocated for eating. Certain individuals opt to conduct the majority of this rapid abstention during the nighttime period while in a state of slumber, subsequently abstaining from food until the subsequent day's lunchtime. To illustrate, in the event that you refrain from consuming food starting from 7 PM the previous evening, you will abstain from eating until 11 AM the following morning. Subsequently, there is a designated time frame of eight hours allocated for consuming meals, followed by the resumption of fasting at 7 PM. Alternatively, you might choose to partake in breakfast and utilize the period between breakfast and early dinner as your designated eating interval, while observing an extended period of fasting during the night and overnight. As an illustration, one could conclude breakfast consumption by 7 AM, proceed to have lunch approximately at noon, and conclude the day with dinner scheduled around 3 PM. Following that, you refrain from consuming any food until 7 AM the subsequent morning. One advantageous aspect of this particular approach lies in the fact that it grants individuals the freedom to selectively determine their eating window, spanning a duration of eight hours, and, in equal measure, decide on a fasting window encompassing a duration of sixteen hours. Should the current arrangement prove excessive, it is permissible to modify the duration of fasting to a period spanning twelve to fourteen hours, accompanied by a widened timeframe designated for consuming meals. This could imply abstaining from eating beyond 7 PM and refraining from doing so until 7 AM the next day, or alternatively, postponing breakfast until 9 AM, allowing for a few hours of delay. By adopting this approach, you can achieve a fasting period of fourteen hours without experiencing excessive discomfort.

The most suitable timings for your schedule can be ascertained by considering your lifestyle, personal preferences, and biological sex. Females generally experience quicker outcomes compared to males, thus a reduced fasting duration may be more advantageous for them, whereas males thrive when following longer time intervals. Provided that you adhere to this prescribed eating schedule for approximately four weeks, it is suggested that you contemplate making further adjustments to it, either by extending the duration or incorporating more days per week.

An additional form of intermittent fasting entails a fasting period of 24 hours. This implies adhering to a specific schedule for meals, such as concluding one's eating period at a designated hour, for instance, midday, and subsequently abstaining from consuming any food until that very hour on the subsequent day. This implies that you will be foregoing dinner on the commencement day and breakfast the following day. In the majority of instances, one typically selects one or two days per week to adhere to this fasting schedule. If you are interested in attempting this approach, I would suggest examining your weekly schedule and identifying a suitable day for a 24-hour fast, as well as determining the specific start and end times for your fasting period. Certain individuals may opt to practice fasting on Mondays due to the demanding nature of the day, which often entails catching up on tasks and responsibilities following the weekend, thereby offering an abundance of diversions. Nevertheless, some individuals perceive Mondays as increasingly burdensome; alternatively, they find solace in Wednesdays due to its position as the midweek, offering respite during times of work-related fatigue. However, certain individuals may perceive a midweek fast as burdensome and disruptive to their productivity. They have a preference for observing the fast during weekends, as these periods tend to offer diminished disturbances and obligations. However, there are individuals who are opposed to imposing limitations on the weekend's liberty. Upon careful examination, it becomes apparent that each day of the week presents both advantages and disadvantages. Accordingly, it is advisable to exercise your judgment and select the option that is most suited to your particular circumstances.

You are permitted to choose your own timeframe for intermittent fasting, encompassing the period between 16 and 24 hours of fasting. If you have already become accustomed to a 16/8 fasting schedule and wish to incorporate a 24-hour fast, consider modifying the fasting window you have already established. One possible rephrase in a formal tone could be: "The progression could be initiated with a ratio of 18 units over 6 units, followed by 20 units over 4 units, and subsequently 22 units over 2 units, until the sum of units totals 24 hours." Consider this as a flexible continuum and framework—allowing you to carefully modify the duration and schedule of your intermittent fasting to suit your individual needs and preferences.

An alternative approach to intermittent fasting, which is often contemplated by many individuals, is the 2/5 method. This pertains to the days on which you are reducing your caloric intake. It is unnecessary to completely eliminate food intake for two days of the week, but it is advisable to significantly reduce consumption during those days. In accordance with standard practice, it is customary to observe two consecutive 24-hour periods each week during which you restrict your calorie intake to a maximum of 600. In this manner, you can still consume nourishment; however, it is imperative that you exercise discernment in selecting your sustenance, ensuring that you achieve a satisfying level of satiety without surpassing your specified caloric objectives. This location offers an excellent opportunity for individuals concerned about discontinuing meals or enduring a full day of fasting initially. One can select a particular day to initiate the reduction of intake, gradually transitioning into the entirety of the fasting duration.

PROCEDURES TO ENGAGE IN INTERMITTENT FASTING

Initial Stage: Comprehend and Make a Choice Regarding the Varieties of Intermittent Fasting

Intermittent fasting comprises a variety of methods that encompass distinct durations for both the periods of eating and the periods of fasting. Today, however, our focus will be directed towards the top five techniques that have endured rigorous scrutiny and experimentation, establishing themselves as the foremost strategies in promoting weight loss.

The 16:8 intermittent fasting protocol, also known as the Leangains method

This type of fasting is well-suited for individuals who typically do not have the opportunity to allocate time for breakfast.

The 16/8 method advocates for a daily fasting period of 16 hours, followed by an eight-hour window for consuming meals (ideally two to three).

This approach posits that restricting one's food consumption to an eight-hour window each day is the optimal and most straightforward strategy for achieving weight loss and weight management. In this scenario, it is necessary to consume the total daily caloric intake within a specific time frame. For example, one could choose to have breakfast and lunch at 10 am, lunch at either 1 pm or 2 pm, and conclude with their final meal by 6 pm.

Should you have any inquiries, please be informed that the quantity of calories or fat consumed during this period holds minimal significance. The principal rationale underlying this dietary approach posits that the prevalent practice of consuming meals over an extended period of up to 16 hours contributes significantly to the prevailing challenges encountered in managing body weight among the majority of individuals.

Although the precise timeframe for experiencing metabolic benefits from intermittent fasting remains uncertain, it is widely acknowledged by experts that refraining from eating for a minimum of 12 hours per day is advantageous, and ideally extending this fasting period to 16 hours is optimal. According to your daily schedule, you have the flexibility to determine when to allocate your eight-hour period. Should you experience hunger, especially in the morning, you may opt to consume your customary breakfast, followed by lunch, and conclude with a minimal meal around 6pm. In this manner, you will retain approximately 12-14 hours of fasting each day, while simultaneously ensuring the intake of calories to prevent enduring prolonged hunger throughout the evening.

Pros

The leangains diet presents an exceptional approach to efficiently develop lean muscle mass, while avoiding the accumulation of any adipose tissue. Additionally, it has been hailed as an effective method for achieving weight reduction and sustaining long-term results. In contrast to alternative protocols of intermittent fasting, the leangains approach involves daily eating habits, thereby eliminating any fasting periods lasting for 24 hours. Consequently, this pattern effectively cultivates a disciplined training routine.

Cons

The leangains approach is characterized by a limited time window, a feature that has been acknowledged as a concern due to its tendency to instill a diet-centric mindset. This would present challenges in adhering to the methodology over an extended duration due to the fundamental fact that it is a dietary regimen.

Similar to numerous other intermittent fasting (IF) approaches, the 16/8 method has encountered scrutiny for disregarding the principle of calories in/calories out. This principle posits that weight loss ensues when the calories consumed do not exceed the calories expended, necessitating adherence to a calorie restriction regimen during the non-fasting periods rather than the indulgence permitted by this method.

Finally, it is a widely held belief that leangains was specifically designed for individuals engaged in bodybuilding, prompting some to contend that optimal outcomes can only be achieved by strictly adhering to the protocol. This necessitates the consumption of appropriate supplements in coordination with the exercise regimen, along with meticulous adherence to specific macronutrient ratios and designated meal timings.

Taking into account all the variables encompassed by the leangains diet, it may necessitate a considerable amount of time to deduce the precise details that will be effective for each individual.

The 5:2 Diet, also known as the Fast Diet

This form of fasting is most suitable for individuals who require a high degree of adaptability.

The 5:2 diet entails a reduction in calorie intake to 25% of energy or calorie requirements on two non-consecutive fasting days, while adhering to a regular eating pattern for the remaining five days of the week.

When observing fasting periods, it is advisable for women to maintain a caloric intake of approximately 500, while men are recommended to consume approximately 600 calories. You have the autonomy to make a selection regarding the two fasting days of the week; however, it is imperative that you allocate at least one non-fasting day in between.

In principle, one adheres to regular eating patterns on the non-fasting days and is free from the need to consider caloric limitations. This implies that due to the overall reduction in calorie consumption throughout the week, it is certain that weight loss will occur.

Suggestion: A recommended strategy for increased efficacy of the diet is to strategically schedule fasting periods on Mondays and Thursdays, during which individuals consume limited portions of two or three meals. On the remaining days, individuals may follow their regular eating patterns.

Pros

The intermittent diet offers a high degree of adaptability. The flexibility offered by this diet plan, which allows individuals to select their fasting days and determine how to distribute their calorie intake (be it during breakfast, lunch, or dinner), ensures that it can be readily accommodated within the schedule of virtually any person.

Additionally, the dietary plan is non-restrictive, in contrast to certain fasting approaches that often impose strict limitations, as it does not impose any prohibitions on specific food items. Therefore, it entails the freedom to consume nutritious meals without any restrictions on specific food choices for a span of five days each week. During the days of fasting, it is essential to prioritize the nutritional value of every bite, ensuring that each morsel contributes to the overall nourishment of the body.

To conclude, the two designated fasting days also serve as an opportunity to cultivate greater mindfulness in meal planning, ensuring the consumption of an appropriate caloric intake.

Cons

Numerous professional nutritionists have expressed doubt regarding the long-term viability of this diet regimen, contending that maintaining rigorous caloric restriction for two days each week indefinitely may pose challenges, especially during occasions such as dining out or holiday festivities.

Additionally, the 5:2 diet presents a significant issue pertaining to the days designated for regular eating. Encouraging individuals to consume anything they desire on the non-fasting days has been characterized as potentially detrimental to weight loss efforts, as it could inadvertently lead to excessive calorie intake. In relation to this matter, nutrition experts have put forth the notion that it is important for one to grasp the fact that consuming food in a manner deemed as 'normal' does not serve as an endorsement to indulge in any and all kinds of food. Consuming a variety of nutritionally deficient foods within your designated eating period may lead to weight gain rather than weight loss.

Finally, adhering to the prescribed low calorie limitation endorsed by the diet necessitates restricting one's food intake, potentially resulting in the exclusion of vital food categories in order to attain the stringent calorie requirement. Ultimately, you may find yourself consuming substandard food in general as you endeavor to restrict your caloric intake.

This issue exacerbates as individuals, including yourself, progressively reduce their fasting frequency due to the accommodating nature of the diet.

Unsweetened Peanut Butter Fudge

1 cup coconut oil

¼ cup unsweetened almond milk

1 cup unsweetened peanut butter

Method

Place peanut butter and coconut oil in the microwave to achieve a softened consistency.

Combine with the remaining ingredients and place them in your blender.

Blend until smooth

Please arrange a baking sheet by interleaving it with parchment paper.

Dispense the mixture onto the surface of the paper.

Chill in the refrigerator for a minimum of three hours, or ideally overnight if feasible.

Your peanut butter fudge is now prepared for consumption. One may prepare a chocolate sauce to enhance the delectable flavor of the dish.

Mix together ¼ cup of unsweetened cocoa powder with 2 tablespoons of coconut oil, then incorporate your preferred sweetening agent. Apply a light drizzle on top of the fudge prior to placing it in the refrigerator.

Ensuring Safety In Physical Activity During Intermittent Fasting

The effectiveness of any weight loss or exercise regimen is contingent upon its long-term sustainability. If your ultimate objective consists of reducing body fat and maintaining your fitness level while practicing intermittent fasting, it is imperative to adhere to a range of safety parameters. Here are some professional insights to assist you in accomplishing that.

Consume a meal in proximity to your exercise session of moderate to high intensity.

This is where the aspect of meal timing becomes relevant. Khorana asserts that the optimal timing of a meal in relation to a moderate- or high-intensity workout is crucial. By doing so, your body will have an accessible source of glycogen reserves to utilize for sustaining your physical exertion.

Stay hydrated

According to Sonpal, it is important to note that fasting does not entail the removal of water. Indeed, he advises increasing your water intake during the fasting period.

Ensure that you maintain proper levels of electrolytes.

According to Sonpal, an excellent source of low-calorie hydration is coconut water. "It effectively restores electrolyte levels, boasts a low caloric content, and possesses a pleasant flavor," he affirms. Gatorade and sports beverages are abundant in sugar, thus it is advisable to limit excessive consumption of these products.

Maintain a reasonably low level of intensity and duration.

If one exerts excessive effort and experiences sensations of dizziness or lightheadedness, it is advised to pause temporarily. It is imperative to pay heed to one's physiological cues.

Take into account the nature of the hurrying.

If you are engaging in a 24-hour intermittent fasting regimen, Lippin advises adhering to low-intensity fitness activities, such as walking, restorative yoga, or gentle pilates. However, when following the 16:8 fasting protocol, a substantial portion of the 16-hour fasting period occurs during the evening, sleep, and early morning, implying that adhering to a specific type of exercise is not of utmost importance.

Pay attention to the signals your body is sending.

It is crucial to pay attention to one's body when engaging in physical activity during intermittent fasting. According to Amenguál, if one begins to experience weakness or dizziness, it is possible that they are encountering low blood sugar levels or dehydration. If that is indeed the circumstance, she advises to promptly choose a carbohydrate-electrolyte beverage and subsequently proceed with the consumption of a nutritionally balanced meal.

While it is true that exercising and practicing intermittent fasting may yield favorable outcomes for certain individuals, it is important to acknowledge that there are others who may not find it amenable or feasible to engage in any form of physical activity during a fasting period. It is advisable to consult with your medical practitioner or healthcare professional prior to commencing any nutritional or physical fitness regimen.

Developing your body into an efficient fat-burning entity

I recommend that you approach this undertaking in a gradual manner, as failing to provide your body with sufficient time to adapt may lead to the temptation of giving up. In order to initiate this, it will be necessary to either eliminate or minimize your carbohydrate consumption to the utmost minimum. When the glycogen stores in your body are depleted, it will utilize your fat reserves as a source of energy. This phenomenon is referred to as ketogenesis. This particular procedure generates ketones within our bloodstream, which are subsequently utilized as a source of energy.

Ketones generate significantly potent energy." or "Ketones yield considerably robust energy. They do not cause fluctuations in our insulin levels.

Several indications that you have transitioned into a state of ketosis include:

You will promptly perceive the distinction once your body successfully acclimates to the metabolic mechanism of burning fat.

You will observe a reinvigorated vitality that has remained dormant for an extended period.

Upon observation, it will become evident that your mind exhibits enhanced clarity and significantly improved levels of concentration.

Lack of somnolence during the mid-afternoon period

You will possess the capability to regulate your physical appetite.

I recommend that you cease the following activities in order to facilitate the transition.

Sugar

Unfavorable developments continue to arise for individuals who have an affinity for incorporating sugar into their dietary preferences. We have taken note of the challenges associated with the impact of sugar on our insulin levels, and as the prevalence of diabetes rises, the resulting physical health complications are also increasingly observed. Sugar can enhance the palatability of food and engender addictive tendencies, nevertheless, it is advisable for all individuals to limit their daily sugar intake to no more than 25 grams, and even less if they currently experience insulin-related complications.

Currently, there is a growing association between sugar consumption and mental health concerns, specifically Alzheimer's disease and other dementia-related issues. These concerns are increasingly apparent in our society, and once we have encountered these challenges, they can prove to be arduous to manage, let alone eradicate. What are the various manners in which an excessive intake of sugar, being a toxic substance for our bodies, can impact our mental well-being? There are indeed multiple ways to approach this matter, and we shall delineate them herein.

The brain and glucose. Certain proponents of sugar have argued that the presence of glucose is essential, as it serves as the primary fuel source for the brain. Certain experts now hold the belief that the brain exclusively relies on glucose due to its limited availability. Consequently, it has been discovered that this reliance results in detrimental effects on both the structure and functioning of the brain.

The genuinely nourishing substances for the brain consist of alternative forms of fuel, notably ketones generated by the body during the digestion of wholesome fats. In a study conducted on a cohort of cognitively sound older individuals, elevated glucose levels were found to be correlated with reduced cognitive capacities, particularly in relation to memory function, along with structural abnormalities observed in the hippocampus region of the brain. The atrophy of the hippocampus is regarded as a prolonged precursor for the onset of Alzheimer's disease.

The connection between the liver, sugar, and its implications on our brain function. A fundamental prerequisite for the optimization of brain functionality lies in the presence of cholesterol, a substance synthesized within the confines of our hepatic organ. The liver performs numerous essential functions, among which processing sugar is particularly noteworthy. By imposing greater demands on the liver's fructose processing capabilities, there is a reduction in the allocation of time and resources for the production of the crucial cholesterol required by the brain.

It is widely acknowledged that the brain possesses significant plasticity, and by consciously selecting a healthy dietary regimen, engaging in regular exercise, and making overall favorable lifestyle choices, it is possible to mitigate numerous age-related issues. However, in engaging in this endeavor, we shall largely assume sole responsibility for upholding the necessary level of discipline. There exists a comprehensive sector that promotes sugar and other processed food items, asserting that these hazardous toxic substances possess beneficial properties.

Additional Hazards Entail

Cardiac Implications - Studies have demonstrated the influence of sugar on the autonomic myocardial activity. G6P, a compound present in regular table sugar, exerts deleterious effects on cardiac tissue at the cellular level.

The consumption of excessive amounts of sugar combined with a sedentary way of life can heighten an individual's vulnerability to the onset of heart failure. Individuals diagnosed with heart failure often succumb to the condition within a span of approximately ten years.

Abdominal adiposity - There has been a concerning escalation in the prevalence of excessive body weight in adolescents and young children over the recent decades. One of the primary factors that has significantly contributed to this prevailing trend is the escalated consumption of fructose. Fructose is a cost-effective variant of sugar employed in carbonated beverages, frozen desserts, baked goods, and even various types of bread.

Fructose appears to enhance the proliferation of visceral adipose tissue, specifically located in our abdominal regions. If a child acquires advanced levels of visceral adipose tissue during early stages of life, there is an increased likelihood of developing obesity in adulthood.

Ravenous Hunger - Our physiques possess inherent mechanisms that signal satiety, indicating the appropriate cessation of eating. Research indicates that sugar has discovered a means to impede those inherent mechanisms. The consumption of food and beverages that are high in sugar is a contributing factor to the development of a physiological condition known as leptin resistance.

When an individual experiences leptin resistance, they fail to experience satiety and feelings of fullness even after consuming moderate amounts of food, leading them to persistently consume excessive quantities of food during each meal.

Our physical systems also encounter difficulty in detecting the presence of sugar within beverages. The human body encounters challenges in effectively signaling the intake of a significant amount of calories from soda or juices due to the distinct way in which this substance is perceived, which differs from the recognition of other forms of food.

Diminishes our innate immunity against bacterial infections (infectious diseases)

Results in the development of cancer

Weakens eyesight

Contributes to the development of hypoglycemia and diabetes" "Induces the occurrence of hypoglycemia and diabetes" "Facilitates the onset of hypoglycemia and diabetes

Causes a rapid increase in adrenaline levels in children.

Contributes to accelerated aging

Aids in the development of obesity.

Exacerbates the likelihood of developing Crohn's disease

Causes arthritis

Causes asthma

Causes gallstones

Leads to the onset of cardiovascular ailments

Causes hemorrhoids

Causes of varicose veins

Reduces production of growth hormones

Increases cholesterol

Disrupts the process of protein absorption

Triggers food allergies

Causes cataracts

The passage of time affects our skin.

Promotes enlargement of our liver and kidneys

Increases tendon fragility.

Triggers instances of cephalalgia and migrainous episodes.

Elevates the vulnerability to acquiring gout.

Has the potential to contribute to the development of Alzheimer's disease.

Causes dizziness

Is addictive

Adverse consequences of discontinuing sugar consumption.

It required approximately one year for me to consciously eliminate sugar from my diet. Once you have experienced that, you will exude abundant vitality without desiring sugary edibles.

When you considerably reduce your sugar consumption, it can lead to a decrease in your blood sugar, subsequently resulting in a variety of symptoms as your body begins to adapt to seeking alternate sources of energy. The typical symptoms experienced by many individuals during sugar withdrawal include nausea, headaches, and fatigue.

Naturally, the severity of your symptoms primarily hinges on the quantity of sugar consumed in your diet prior to this. If you previously consumed a larger proportion of sugary candies and sweet treats, you are more prone to encountering these symptoms compared to when sugar made up only a minimal portion of your diet.

"Some of the most frequently observed symptoms resulting from the abstention of sugar include:

Headaches

Bloating

Nausea

Muscle aches

Diarrhea

Fatigue

Hunger

Anxiety

Depression

Cravings

Chills

Stages of Sugar Withdrawal

Even though the catalogue of prevalent adverse reactions might seem overwhelming, it is important to bear in mind that these symptoms are transient and typically subside within a few days for the majority of individuals. Presented below are the sequential phases that one can anticipate upon adopting the decision to eliminate sugar from their dietary intake:

1. Feeling Motivated

When an individual chooses to eliminate sugar from their diet, they are likely to experience a significant surge in motivation and become prepared to enjoy the positive outcomes associated with adopting a healthier dietary and lifestyle approach. Keep it up, as you'll need this motivation to propel you through the cravings, headaches and fatigue yet to come.

2. Cravings Commence to Emerge

Cravings constitute one of the primary indicators of sugar withdrawal during its early stages. Numerous individuals, for example, adhere to a predetermined schedule regarding their dietary choices, and may discover themselves casting a brief gaze at the vending machine once the hunger pangs begin to manifest in the mid-morning.

Throughout this stage, it is recommended to be proactive by ensuring the availability of nutritious snacks, thereby enhancing the ability to resist the temptation of indulging in preferred confections.

3. Symptoms Peak

Shortly after the onset of cravings, you may commence experiencing some of the aforementioned symptoms associated with sugar withdrawal. Headaches, hunger, chills, and even experiencing diarrhea due to sugar withdrawal can emerge, rendering it increasingly challenging to sustain motivation.

Recall the rationale behind your initial decision to adopt a more nutritious dietary regimen, and employ that as a source of motivation to persevere resolutely along the trajectory towards enhanced well-being.

4. You commence to experience an improvement in your well-being.

Once your symptoms begin to dissipate, you are apt to experience an improved state of well-being. Numerous individuals have documented enhancements in their skin condition, diminished cognitive impairments, and an elevated vitality status through the cessation of the consumption of additional sugar.

Additionally, by adhering to a wholesome dietary regimen and incorporating a greater proportion of nutrient-rich foods into your daily routine, you will decrease your susceptibility to chronic ailments and experience enhanced overall well-being.

Methods for mitigating or curbing the desire for sugar

In the beginning, refrain from entirely eliminating sugar from your diet. Although it might be enticing to eliminate everything at once, this approach is undoubtedly a recipe for surrendering and experiencing a relapse. Instead, I suggest gradually eliminating one or two sugary foods from your dietary intake. If you have a preference for soda, cookies, and a nightly bowl of ice cream, it is advisable to select one item at a time and seek out a more nutritious substitute. Rather than consuming soda, consider substituting it with fruit tea or water infused with a hint of fruit juice. If you possess an appreciation for cookies, I suggest engaging in the process of their creation or perhaps opting for the consumption of fruit as an alternative. If you find yourself pondering the potential absence of your habitual evening consumption of ice cream, I would encourage you to consider partaking in a modest portion of organic dark chocolate as an alternative. With such substitutions, you will gradually discover an increased level of convenience in effectively controlling your sugar cravings, thereby avoiding reliance on processed confections.

Once you have commenced the regulation or eradication of explicit sugars from your dietary regimen, it is imperative to commence an investigation into the concealed sugars that elude your awareness. Develop a practice of carefully reviewing the label of each item you acquire. It may astound you to discover that numerous food products incorporate sugar or corn syrup within their composition, even if they do not inherently possess sweetness.

Deliberately opting to acquire food items devoid of additional sugars is a commendable strategy to overcome one's yearning for sugar and diminish the overall intake of this sweet substance.

If one continues to experience a persistent desire for sugar, the subsequent course of action to consider would be engaging in a diversionary activity. Engaging in rigorous physical activity can effectively divert your attention from cravings for sugary substances. In addition, engaging in supplementary physical activity induces the release of endorphins, which replicate the pleasurable sensation experienced from consuming sugary substances, albeit in a nourishing manner. In addition to this, the majority of individuals are hesitant to negate the calorie-burning benefits of an intense exercise session by consuming a container of high-fat ice cream.

Lastly, it is imperative to allocate some time for oneself. Please grant yourself the indulgence of consuming one portion of a nutritious and well-balanced confection on a daily basis. This could consist of a portion of organic dark chocolate, a petite serving of natural ice cream, or even a piece of fruit that you have been reserving. Reinforcing the thought that a reward awaits you in your place of residence can serve as a highly effective strategy for incentivizing oneself to combat the sugar cravings that persist while navigating through one's everyday obligations.

Reducing insulin resistance

Type 2 diabetes is a prevalent form of diabetes that can be effectively managed through the implementation of this dietary plan. In this particular ailment, there is an elevation in blood sugar levels along with the presence of insulin resistance within the body. Any intervention that aids in decreasing insulin resistance will contribute to the reduction of blood glucose levels within the body. Numerous studies have demonstrated that intermittent fasting effectively mitigates insulin resistance within the human body. A conducted study on rats with diabetes has revealed that fasting assists in safeguarding them against kidney damage and the accompanying complications associated with diabetes.

Helps in reducing inflammation

Prolonged exposure to oxidative stress can contribute significantly to the acceleration of aging processes and the development of various chronic ailments. This phenomenon arises when volatile molecules undergo reaction with essential molecules such as protein or DNA, thereby inflicting harm upon them in the course of the reaction. Multiple research studies have demonstrated that intermittent fasting effectively enhances the body's resilience against oxidative stress.

It is beneficial for cardiovascular health.

Heart disease is a pernicious issue afflicting the human race. The majority of health indicators are correlated with an escalation or reduction in the risk linked to cardiovascular ailments. Intermittent fasting contributes to the enhancement of multiple risk factors such as blood pressure, high-density lipoprotein cholesterol, triglyceride levels, and the regulation of blood glucose levels. Nevertheless, the bulk of the data substantiating these assertions

have been gathered from research conducted on animals.
Enhances cardiac well-being Augments the health of your cardiovascular system Enhances the overall well-being of your heart

There exist various health indicators that can provide insight into whether one is potentially at a risk. The aforementioned markers encompass indicators such as arterial pressure, serum cholesterol levels, blood triglyceride levels, and blood glucose levels. Intermittent fasting contributes to the enhancement of all these health factors. Based on your personal caloric intake and fasting regimen, you are likely to observe a favorable improvement in the health of your cardiovascular system.
Stimulates the cellular repair process.

Upon initiation of the fasting period, the body's cells commence the systemic elimination of waste products. This procedure entails the degradation of dysfunctional cells and proteins contained within it. The elimination of waste is commonly known as autophagy. An augmentation of autophagy confers added safeguarding against malignancy and ailments such as Alzheimer's. It aids in the elimination of accumulated cellular waste.

Intermittent fasting can also contribute to the enhancement of one's overall well-being and prolongation of life expectancy. Incorporating a straightforward dietary regimen yields numerous advantages for one's overall well-being. By adhering to the intermittent diet, you will have the capability to accomplish your health and weight loss objectives.

Chapter Seven: Strategies for Suppressing Hunger Throughout the Period of Fasting

Provided that you possess human physiology and engaged in the practice of intermittent fasting, it is inevitable that you will experience periods of hunger at some juncture. Several methods for managing hunger include: "

Consuming copious amounts of water Hydrating sufficiently

In addition to being the most healthy and convenient approach to combating hunger, maintaining proper hydration can greatly facilitate the process of fasting. Frequently, the sensation of thirst is mistaken for hunger, thus whenever you experience feelings of hunger, simply consume a glass of water promptly. Please take note of this, as it will be your primary method to prevent hunger.

Please partake in a serving of either coffee or organic tea.

In addition to water, alternative liquids can aid in mitigating hunger sensations effectively. Caffeine and other substances that activate the central nervous system function as agents that reduce appetite. It has been scientifically established that the consumption of coffee leads to the stimulation of cholecystokinin (CCK) hormone release, which is one of the hormones discharged post-meal, inducing a sensation of tranquility. This hormone induces satiety and suppresses the sensation of hunger.

Furthermore, partaking in a modest beverage such as tea or coffee can enhance your vitality while providing the added benefit of supplying an influx of antioxidant properties. Commence your day by indulging in a beverage of your choice, be it tea or coffee, or avail yourself of a cup at your discretion when hunger pangs emerge, ideally prior to breaking your fast.

Meditation

Meditation facilitates relaxation, fosters mental composure, and enables deliberate regulation of cognitive processes. This can facilitate the regulation of anxiety and stress levels. Despite its difficulty, meditation yields remarkable results in suppressing hunger over an extended period. With improved proficiency, one will acquire the skill to manage appetite and potentially even come to embrace it.

Engaging in meditation will enable you to resist the allure of breaking a fast by facilitating clear and focused contemplation on your desires and the advantageous outcomes that await you through steadfast adherence to your fasting regimen.

Participate in brief and vigorous physical activity.

Incorporating brief and vigorous exercise sessions amidst the fasting period is an effective strategy to divert one's thoughts away from hunger. Intense physical activity, such as engaging in sprints or engaging in weight lifting exercises, has the capacity to effectively reduce body fat, enhance muscle growth, and notably, directly decrease one's appetite.

Various forms of physical activity can result in the generation or diminishment of diverse varieties of hormones that aid in suppressing appetite. An example would be aerobic exercises, which have been found to inhibit the hormone ghrelin, a known appetite stimulant, while simultaneously promoting the production of peptide YY, an appetite suppressant.

If you are not present at your place of employment, it is recommended that you engage in the diligent completion of domestic tasks.

If your designated fasting day coincides with a non-working day (or a day wherein you are stationed at home without work obligations), engaging in household chores can effectively alleviate hunger pangs.

Engaging in the tasks of cleaning or gardening can divert your attention away from the consumption of food, while concurrently assisting in the creation of a well-ordered and pristine outdoor space. Furthermore, you have the opportunity to capitalize on this advantage and cultivate your own sustenance. Locally cultivated sustenance presents the optimal means to maintain a nutritious lifestyle while circumventing potential exposure to unfamiliar contaminants.

Are there any outstanding work-related tasks?

Are you aware of the report or project that you have been deferring, or the multitude of unread emails that are accumulating in your inbox? This offers a remarkable opportunity to address and focus on these areas. We kindly request that you ensure the maximization of productivity during your fasting period, refraining from excessive preoccupation with anticipation for the forthcoming meal.

In periods of abstinence from eating, direct your attention towards other meaningful pursuits such as academic endeavors, professional obligations, or engaging in socially relevant activities. The more occupied you are, the greater the likelihood of achieving success in your fasting endeavors.

Participate in athletic activities or pursue a recreational pastime.

Engaging in any form of physical activity will yield beneficial effects on your physique, provided it is maintained at a moderate level. If you possess a preferred sport such as basketball, tennis, or any other sort of physical pastime like boxing, we encourage you to partake in it throughout the fasting period.

This method presents a commendable approach to attaining the dual objectives of physical exercise and fasting, as it effectively directs one's mental attention towards the activity at hand, rather than fixating on the aspects of abstaining from food or engaging in exercise. This is because it is an activity that brings you pleasure and you perceive it as leisurely recreation.

Take a walk

Engaging in brisk walks enhances the fat-burning benefits associated with a rapid pace. Engaging in a brisk walk also enhances cardiovascular health and fosters overall well-being. Engaging in a fusion of a swift pace and a brisk stride would likely yield optimal benefits for your physical well-being.

Similar to other forms of physical activity, engaging in a brisk walk can help regulate your appetite. It achieves this by initially offering an enjoyable diversion, thereby stimulating the body to initiate the process of utilizing stored fat as a source of energy.

One could engage in activities such as walking the dog, running errands to purchase groceries, or opting to commute on foot to the workplace instead of relying on public transportation, particularly during morning hours.

Consume a variety of nourishments

This ought to be considered as the final recourse for managing hunger. In the instance where one discovers that complete control over their hunger is not attainable and they are truly compelled to consume food, the most suitable course of action would be to engage in a "controlled fast" akin to the phase of moderated food intake observed in the Warrior Diet methodology.

During your fast, it will be necessary for you to consume small portions of food. Consume foods that exhibit a minimal glycemic index, thereby minimizing any potential impact on your blood glucose levels. The diet composition ought to exclusively consist of vegetables and fruits, with no allowance for any form of cooking. Additionally, ensure that the portions are kept modest.

Variations in Patterns of Interruption and Cessation of Consumption

Although the fundamental principles underlying the various approaches to intermittent fasting remain consistent, there exist a multitude of divergent methods to pursue this dietary practice. The most advisable course of action would be to experiment with a few alternatives, observing and considering which one elicits the most favorable and effortless response from your body.

16:8 Method

This approach entails a fasting period of 16 hours for men and 14 hours for women, followed by the consumption of an appropriate quantity of calories during the remaining 8 to 10 hours. Throughout this duration, it is advised to exclusively partake in comestibles devoid of any caloric content, such as black coffee (a touch of cream is permissible), water, artificially sweetened beverages, and gum that is free of sugar. The most straightforward approach to implement this timetable would be to refrain from consuming any food after the evening meal, allowing for a fasting period of 14 to 16 hours thereafter. This entails forgoing breakfast and acquiring sustenance in the early afternoon.

Once more, the exact timing of your fasting is of relatively minor significance compared to the imperative of consistently fasting for an equivalent duration. If one's fasting period is subject to significant variations, it may result in an inconsistent modulation of hormonal levels, thereby hindering the body's ability to effectively lose any superfluous weight, among other implications. In the event that you are unable to allocate sufficient time to consume a complete meal to conclude the fasting period in the customary manner, it is imperative that you, at the very least, partake in some form of sustenance to maintain your body's adherence to the appropriate rhythm.

If you are exercising, as well as intermittently fasting, it is important to ensure that you are eating more carbohydrates than fats while you are working out, while on days you are not exercising the opposite is true. It is imperative to maintain a consistent level of protein intake on a daily basis. Make an effort to avoid consuming processed foods whenever feasible.

One notable advantage of this fasting regimen is its exceptional adaptability, enabling it to effectively accommodate a diverse range of schedules. The majority of individuals tend to derive benefit by opting for either two substantial meals within the designated 8 or 10-hour feeding window, or dividing that allocated time into three smaller meal portions, as it aligns with the innate programming of the general populace.

When engaging in both exercise and fasting, it is crucial to consistently commence the fast with a combination of protein, vegetables, and fruit. If you typically engage in physical exercise immediately following the cessation of your fasting period, it is imperative to ensure an adequate intake of carbohydrates in order to provide your muscles with the necessary energy for maximizing the efficacy of your workout.

If you intend to engage in physical activity, it is generally advisable to commence the early afternoon by consuming a nourishing meal of moderate caloric content. Subsequently, engage in physical activity no later than three hours prior to consuming a substantial meal thereafter. In this more substantial dining occasion, it is crucial to incorporate a greater quantity of complex carbohydrates. It is permissible to indulge in a small dessert, as long as it is consumed in moderation. Please bear in mind that fasting should not be equated with engaging in a dietary regimen.

It is crucial to make appropriate adjustments to your caloric intake on days when you do not intend to engage in physical exercise. Commence by reducing your consumption of carbohydrates, while emphasizing the inclusion of ample protein, dark green, leafy vegetables, and moderate portions of fruit. In contrast to the days when you engage in physical activity, it is recommended that the initial meal consumed on days of rest should constitute the highest caloric intake. Specifically, this particular meal should account for approximately 40 percent of your daily caloric requirement.

Please bear in mind that throughout this meal, it is advisable to consume a greater proportion of protein relative to other nutrients. When considering your last meal before your period of rest, it is essential to incorporate a protein-rich food that requires lengthy digestion. This will not only provide sustained satiety, but also extend the duration of the fasting period the next morning. Additionally, it furnishes the body with an ample supply of stored amino acids, which serves to safeguard against muscle degradation during the fasting period.

Eat-Stop-Eat

This particular fasting method can be regarded as highly advantageous for individuals who are already consuming a nutritious diet but are seeking to further enhance their weight loss results. In this particular program, individuals refrain from consuming any food for one or two days per week. Throughout this time frame, it is advised to limit your consumption to items that possess negligible caloric value. This can include black coffee with a small amount of cream, water, sugar-free soft drinks, and gum without sugar.

Once the fasting period is concluded, it is imperative to exercise restraint in consuming excessive quantities of food beyond one's usual intake. It is highly advisable to avoid engaging in episodes of excessive eating, as prolonged cycles of fasting and bingeing can have detrimental effects on one's physical well-being. Consistently, it is crucial to exercise restraint and discipline in order to maximize the benefits of the fasting period.

The rapid cycle operates under the premise that in order to achieve a weekly weight loss of one pound, one must simply abstain from a total of 3,500 calories. Thus, it would be advisable to expeditiously address the matter in two swift intervals rather than refraining from consumption for a fraction of each day. This fasting regimen prioritizes resistance weight training to optimize its advantages.

It may initially pose a challenge for individuals to abstain from eating for a whole day, however, it is entirely permissible to gradually acclimate oneself to this practice by gradually extending the duration of abstinence and incrementally building up one's fasting endurance through repeated experience. An effective strategy is to commence by selecting days in which you are aware of the absence of any pre-existing gastronomic commitments. Commencing a fasting regimen on a day when one is aware of a scheduled lunch meeting is an ill-advised course of action.

When commencing this rapid cycle for the first time, it is common to experience fatigue, headaches, or feelings of anger or anxiousness. These effects can be regarded as indicators to pause the current fast, as they are commonly observed side-effects. The aforementioned adverse effects will diminish over time as your body acclimates to the new menstrual cycle.

Following a prolonged period of caloric deprivation for an entire day, it is quite normal to experience an inclination to engage in excessive eating during your initial meal. It is imperative that you possess the necessary discipline to resist these impulses, as indulging in such behavior is not only detrimental to your well-being, but it has the potential to negate all the diligent efforts you have put forth in the preceding 24 hours. Exhibit self-control and ensure that your fasting endeavors yield significant results.

"The Dietary Regimen of a Warrior

The Warrior Diet enhances the 16:8 Program by advocating for a fasting period of approximately 20 hours daily, followed by a single meal consuming the entirety of your daily caloric intake within the remaining four-hour window.

This particular variant of intermittent fasting is based on the principle that humans possess an innate tendency to consume food during the nighttime hours. Hence, consuming food during nighttime facilitates the body's efficient assimilation of essential nutrients. In this instance, the term "fasting" may not accurately represent the practice being described, as it permits the consumption of a portion of uncooked produce or fruits, as well as a possible portion of protein, if one finds it difficult to abstain from eating entirely.

This mechanism is effective as it elicits the activation of the body's inherent sympathetic nervous system, thereby inducing a fight or flight response. Consequently, this response enhances innate alertness levels, augments energy, and concurrently elevates the rate of fat metabolism. The substantial dinner served every night enables the body to dedicate its resources to the process of self-repair and muscular enhancement. When adhering to the Warrior Diet, it is imperative to commence each nocturnal repast with a serving of vegetables, subsequently succeeded by the inclusion of protein, fat, and carbohydrates.

This particular method of fasting is widely embraced due to two primary factors. Initially, the inclusion of a limited selection of modest and permissible snacks throughout the fasting procedure adds appeal to individuals embarking on this practice for the first time. Moreover, the majority of individuals who engage in this particular type of fasting consistently observe a noteworthy surge in their energy levels throughout the day, coupled with a noticeable augmentation in the rate of weekly fat loss.

However, the somewhat rigorous character of this dietary regimen may pose challenges for individuals attempting to adhere to it over extended durations. The scheduling of the substantial meal can pose a challenge for certain individuals to adhere to, as it has the potential to intrude upon various social commitments. Lastly, there are individuals who express discontent towards the idea of being obligated to consume their meals in a particular sequence. Engage in a personal experiment and ascertain which approach yields desirable outcomes for your circumstances.

Sustainable Weight Reduction

This particular approach to intermittent fasting integrates components from various other fasting styles, resulting in a highly distinctive method. Fortunately, you are granted a designated day each week where you have the opportunity to deviate from your prescribed regimen. Unfortunately, there is an unfavorable aspect to this, as it entails a subsequent period of fasting lasting one and a half days, followed by a distribution of fasting intervals between the 16:8 and 20:4 methods for the remaining days of the week.

It is imperative to arrange periods of exercise cessation during the latter segment of the 36-hour cycle in order to adhere to this diet plan. Alternatively, it is essential to remain occupied during these periods to effectively counteract your hunger. If you encounter difficulties in managing your food cravings during scheduled indulgence days, this particular method of intermittent fasting may not be suitable for you, as it necessitates a rapid and regular transition from a high intake to a minimal consumption of food.

Furthermore, it is imperative to refrain from attempting to endure a span of 36 hours without the consumption of nourishment in one sitting. It is essential to gradually enhance your body's capacity to endure prolonged periods of fasting. Therefore, it is generally advisable to commence with an alternative form of intermittent fasting and gradually progress towards the Fat Loss Forever approach once your body has already ceased its accustomed pattern of consuming meals every three or four hours.

Please bear in mind the importance of observing responsible fasting practices, and refraining from exerting yourself to the extent that it leads to physical discomfort. Furthermore, it is crucial to maintain a regular fasting schedule in order to provide your body with the necessary adaptation period.

Intermittent Fasting Diet

This method of intermittent fasting essentially allows you to avoid prolonged periods without food, should you desire. On alternating days, you adhere to a regular eating pattern, while on the remaining days, you only ingest one-fifth of the calories you typically consume. The mean daily caloric intake ranges from 2,000 to 2,500 calories, thereby indicating that the average non-working day fluctuates between 400 and 500 calories. If one derives pleasure from engaging in daily physical activity, this particular approach to intermittent fasting may not be suitable, as it necessitates significant reduction in workout intensity during non-fasting periods.

When initially pursuing this method of intermittent fasting, facing the low-calorie days can be facilitated by opting for any of several protein shakes available as a viable solution. It is essential to transition back to authentic, whole foods during these periods, as they consistently provide superior nutritional benefits compared to meal replacement shakes.

This variant of intermittent fasting primarily focuses on achieving weight loss. Individuals who attempt this method typically achieve an average weight loss rate of approximately two to three pounds per week. When embarking on the Alternate Day Diet, it is of utmost importance to adhere to a consistent eating pattern on your full-calorie days. Engaging in excessive consumption not only undermines any achievements you have accomplished, but it can also inflict severe harm upon your physical well-being if prolonged.

Not adhering to regular meal patterns.

If you possess a curiosity regarding the advantages of intermittent fasting and find yourself with an inconsistent timetable or uncertainty about its suitability, partaking in the occasional omission of a meal or two might be the variant of intermittent fasting that aligns with your needs. As previously mentioned, establishing a regular fasting regimen is crucial for achieving optimal outcomes through concerted effort. Nevertheless, it should be noted that intermittent fasting also offers certain advantages in certain instances.

Furthermore, upon experiencing occasional meal omission, one can personally witness the simplicity of the practice, thereby paving the way for subsequent transformative adjustments. Given the abundance of intermittent fasting options currently accessible, there is a high probability that one of them will align with your schedule. Therefore, it would be advisable to consider giving it a try. What potential detriments do you have to consider (apart from shedding a few pounds)?